Ayurveda Diet

Ayurveda Diet Tips for Healthy Living and Weight Loss

The information herein is offered for informational purposes solely, and is universal as so. The presentation of the information is without contract or any type of guarantee assurance.

The trademarks that are used are without any consent, and the publication of the trademark is without permission or backing by the trademark owner. All trademarks and brands within this book are for clarifying purposes only and are the owned by the owners themselves, not affiliated with this document.

Table of Contents

Introduction

I want to thank you and congratulate you for downloading the book, *"Ayurveda Diet: Ayurveda Diet Tips for Healthy Living and Weight Loss."*

This book contains proven steps and strategies on how to become healthier, happier and better looking by following the Ayurveda diet and the principles behind it.

Have you ever tried losing weight, only to be unsuccessful in your efforts? Do you want to achieve optimum health? The book, which is based on the principles of the ancient Indian traditional medicinal system called Ayurveda, offers you a new way of dealing with the way you eat. The book also offers insights and tips on how to eat well.

Furthermore, it shatters your perceptions of what healthy eating should be. As you learn the Ayurveda diet principles, you will realize that you are actually doing it all wrong. You will also be armed with the knowledge that will help you achieve a healthy weight correctly.

Thanks again for downloading this book, I hope you enjoy it!

Chapter 1: What is Ayurveda?

Ayurveda has been around for over five millennia. It is a natural healing system with origins in India's Vedic culture. While not openly practiced in India during the period of foreign occupation, the system has been revived in many parts of the world and in its homeland. Both traditional Chinese and Tibetan medicine have Ayurveda roots. Even ancient Greek medicine adopted concepts described originally in Ayurveda medical texts that date back to several millennia.

Ayurveda is a life science (*Ayur* is life, *Veda* is knowledge or science). More than just a system to treat illness, it offers wisdom meant to help people realize their full potential and stay on top of their game. Ayurveda – while giving guidelines on ideal seasonal and daily routines, behavior, the right use of the senses, and diet – reminds people that health is the dynamic and balanced integration between the body, mind, spirit and environment.

As human beings belong to nature, Ayurveda has three basic energies or *doshas* that govern their outer and inner environments - structure, transformation and movement. In Sanskrit, they are known as kapha (earth), pitta (fire), and vata (wind). The fundamental forces are responsible for the characteristics of your body and mind.

Everyone has a unique proportion of the 3 forces that mold their nature. When kapha is dominant, you tend to be methodical, easy-going, and nurturing. If pitta dominates, you tend to be goal-oriented, intelligent and intense, and have a strong desire for life. If vata dominates, you tend to be changeable, energetic, enthusiastic, light and thin.

While many people have all the three forces, most have one or two dominating forces. There is an imbalance-and-balanced expression for every element. When kapha is balanced, a person is stable, supportive and sweet, but when it is imbalanced, he may experience sinus congestion, weight gain and sluggishness.

When pitta is balanced, a person is friendly, warm and disciplined. He can also be a good speaker and leader, but when imbalance, he may become irritable, compulsive, and may suffer from an inflammatory condition or indigestion. When vata is balanced, a person may be creative and lively, but when it is not balanced, he may experience constipation, difficulty focusing, dry skin, insomnia, and anxiety.

A vital Ayurveda goal is to know your ideal balance state and when you are out of balance. It also aims to offer interventions through aromatherapy, herbs, music, massage treatments, meditation, and even diet to reestablish balance.

Determining Dosha Type

Many websites and books on Ayurveda offer questionnaires that are useful in determining your body/mind constitution. Many of the questionnaires are similar and will also give similar results. Also, know that short questionnaires will give a more approximate and general result. Your body also changes with seasons, life situations and age, thus, there is a great possibility that the results will change. Taking various questionnaires will offer you a more specific dosha type result.

Moreover, the dosha types exhibit various characteristics like:

Vata

- Naturally creative
- Light build
- Prefer humid, warm climates
- Sensitive
- Dry skin

Pitta

- Irritable
- Fair skin
- Prefer cold climates
- Hard-working, productive
- Muscular, medium build

Kapha

- Methodical, stable
- Heavy build
- Prefer dry, warm climates
- Oily skin
- Easygoing

Ayurveda and Diet

While this book is about Ayurveda, it centers more on the Ayurveda diet and how it can benefit your health and help you lose weight. When you know your dosha type, you should strive to follow the lifestyle routine and diet that is specific for your body/mind composition. If you are mostly vata, for example, you should eat more warm and cooked foods. Also, you need to avoid iced drinks, and add warming spices like ginger, cloves and cinnamon to your meals.

The following chapters will discuss more on the Ayurveda diet, its health benefits, how it can help you lose weight, what foods to buy for your dosha type, and other food-related guidelines. Read on and know how the Ayurveda diet can immensely improve your health and help you lose weight.

Chapter 2: The Ayurveda Diet

When it comes to the Ayurveda diet, you don't have to think that you'll be constantly eating only vegetables, rice and legumes. The diet's fundamental principles are applicable to any cuisine, be it Asian, Mediterranean, European, or any other cuisine.

The saying 'You are what you eat' holds true on a physical and psychological level. When your diet mostly consists of French fries and hamburgers, you may probably feel like French fries and hamburgers – and not in a good way. In the Ayurveda diet, it is essential that your foods are fresh, organic, local and seasonal. However, fresh doesn't always mean 'raw'. What you should consume are whole, freshly-cooked meals.

Cook more often with fresh produce. Use some of the basic Ayurveda spices like coriander, cumin, ginger and turmeric. You can add the spices to any dish that you cook. Aside from being excellent digestion and flavor enhancers, Ayurveda spices can also offer medicinal benefits.

Benefits of the Ayurveda Diet

Ailment Cure. The Ayurveda principles state that to cure all health-related problems, it is crucial to change the patient's diet. The combination of Ayurveda dietary rules and the right supplements is believed to cure any health issue.

Healthy Weight. The Ayurveda diet can help you achieve a healthy and normal weight – without getting too thin. Many contemporary weight loss plans and fads damage the body by depleting or burning nutrients – not only excess fat. The Ayurveda diet promotes eating foods according to a person's dosha. Additionally, individuals suffering from anorexia can also use the Ayurveda diet to be healthier.

Increased Life Span. When you follow the Ayurveda diet, you achieve balance among the doshas. You can expect your mind and body to function at their best. The diet also helps to create new cells and enhances your existing cells' survival period. When your cells function efficiently, you live a healthier and longer life.

Increased Energy. In Ayurveda, the digestive system is believed to be the body's main energy source. The first effect is on your digestive system as you eat. After achieving balance, your body's energy blocks are released, thereby ensuring a better energy flow.

Personalized for your Dietary Needs. The Ayurveda is based on the six tastes, including astringent, bitter, sour, salty, sweet and pungent. It's also based on the six food qualities like heavy/light, hot/cold, and oily/dry. Some of the tastes and qualities increase any of the three doshas (vata, pitta, and kapha), while others work in decreasing them.

Each person's diet varies accordingly, and you are free to choose any food according to the qualities and tastes. It is easier for you to manage it then, and you have a number of foods to choose from.

<u>Reduces Ama</u>. In Ayurveda, the term 'ama' means toxicity, which works against 'agni.' When your 'agni' (digestive fire) is low, your body is not capable of properly digesting food. This leads to ama (toxin) production in your body.

Six Tastes in the Ayurveda Diet

Ayurveda distinguishes six tastes and you should have all of them in your everyday diet. They are:

1. Sweet – milk, pasta, rice, honey, sugar, etc.

2. Sour – vinegar, yogurt, hard cheese, lemons, etc.

3. Salty – salt or any food that contains salt

4. Pungent – ginger, cayenne, chili peppers, any hot spice

5. Bitter – lettuce, turmeric, leafy greens, etc.

6. Astringent – lentils, beans, pomegranate, etc.

The six tastes are in the order that your body digests them. Any sweets or carb dish you eat gets digested first, thus, it is advisable to eat your dessert at the beginning of your meal. On the other hand, you need to eat salad as you end your meal.

Integrating all the six tastes in the Ayurveda diet contributes to a feeling of fullness at the end of each meal. As such, cravings are usually caused by not having the six tastes in your meals. A lot of people often omit the astringent and bitter tastes, even when both tastes are important. When you are eating something astringent or bitter at the end of your meal, you reduce your craving to eat desserts.

In the Ayurveda diet, integrating the six tastes improves your health immensely. You also get to lose some unwanted weight effortlessly

Agni

In the Ayurveda diet, agni (digestive fire) is considered the most important concept by Ayurveda practitioners and physicians. You can digest whatever you consume when your agni is strong and healthy. When your digestive fire is weak, you are unable to digest your food and your body easily produces toxins.

For agni balance, try to eat lightly and follow some healthy eating habits. You may include ginger tea in your diet. Peel and grate ¼ inch of ginger. Pour hot water over it and allow it to sit for 5 minutes. Sip the tea daily.

Eating Out

The practice of eating outside the home is prevalent throughout the world, especially if you don't want to cook your own meals or if you don't have the time to prepare your meals after work. However, you can still follow the Ayurveda diet as long as you know some basic tips when it comes to dining out.

The first and important pointer on eating out is to ask for warm or room temperature water, instead of cold water with lots of ice. Nothing kills the agni (digestive fire) faster than drinking cold water on an empty stomach.

Keep in mind the quality and tastes of food when you dine out. If you are armed with the knowledge on what qualities and tastes balance your Ayurveda body type, you can make the right food choices.

If your dosha is predominantly pitta, you will do fine if you eat at salad bars and eat mostly raw food. You may also eat vegetarian dishes. Avoid eating tomato, garlicky and deep fried dishes. Know that anything spicy/hot aggravates pitta.

If your dosha is predominantly vata, it is best to favor warm soup over a cold salad. When dining out, avoid cold, raw foods and concentrate more on warm, well-cooked dishes.

If your dosha is predominantly kapha, you should do well to eat light food items like light vegetarian dishes and lightly cooked/steamed vegetables. Avoid dishes that are oily/heavy and those that are fried and have lots of sour cream or cheese.

Healthy Eating Habits

If you take note of some healthy habits and favor healthy foods for your dominant dosha, you can augment your digestion and experience immense health benefits.

- Eating should be a cherished ritual. Before eating, say grace or take three to five slow breaths. Such process can prepare you to receive food.

- Eat food that is lovingly prepared. The cook's energy is in the food, therefore, you need to avoid eating dishes made by a resentful cook. In Ayurveda, not only do you eat food, you also take in the cook's emotions.

- Eat in a calm place. Don't eat with the radio or television turned on. Don't even read. Also, engage in limited conversation and don't talk about emotionally intense subject matters.

- Chew your food well. As you eat, be mindful of the food in your mouth. Properly chewing your food improves absorption and digestion.

- Eat with a moderate pace until you are three-quarters full. One of society's major disease causes is overeating. As you eat a lot of food, your digestion suffers. After you have finished eating, you should no longer feel hungry and heavy.

- Don't drink a lot of liquids with your meals. Half a cup of room temp water is acceptable. You don't have to drink liquids with moist meals. However, in eating dry meals, you may need to drink more. Take all your drinks, including water, warm or at room temperature as cold drinks decrease digestion by destroying the digestive fire.

- Allow 15 to 20 minutes to digest your food. After eating your meal, rest a bit and allow your food to digest before doing other things. By this, read a book or have a conversation with your eating companion. You can also take a walk. Take at least three to five breaths as a culmination of your meal.

- Let your meals digest for at least three hours. This means, you can take 3 to 5 meals a day.

- Make lunch as your heaviest meal. The smallest should be your dinner. Your body digests food best at around lunchtime when the sun is high. The rhythm of the body mirrors the universe's rhythm. Also, you need to eat breakfast. Eat a larger breakfast if you are famished. If not, drink ginger tea as an appetite stimulate, so you can have even a small breakfast.

While losing excess fat and normalizing body weight is a great side effect of following the Ayurveda diet, it is even more important to know that Ayurveda's goal is to bring you back to your true constitution. It is also important to restore balance in your mind and body. Ayurveda takes you back to your real nature where you experience happiness, balance and optimal health.

Chapter 3: Foods to Eat for your Dosha

Depending on your dosha, know what foods are right for you. As you know your Ayurveda body type (vata, pitta, and kapha), you will find out what foods you should eat.

Vata benefits from warm, oily and heavy food. Such qualities are important, and are more relevant than the individual foods. Some of the best vata foods are:

- Warm milk – Preferably, drink it with a pinch of cardamom and powdered ginger.
- Butter or clarified butter (ghee) - You can add it to any food item.
- Ginger (fresh) - It's considered the best pungent spice. You can also make ginger tea or add ginger to your meals.
- Cream of wheat or rice - You can add ginger, cardamom and ghee to it.
- Almonds - Use boiling water to rinse them then remove the skin. Slightly roast the almonds in ghee.
- Root vegetables like sweet potatoes, red beets, and carrots - You can cook and spice them up.
- Sweet fruit - Examples are red grapes, figs and dates - It's best to eat room temperature fruits. Soak dried fruits first before eating them.
- Chicken broth
- Kichari - You can pair it with root vegetables, fresh ginger and ghee.

Pitta benefits from dry, cold and heavy foods. Examples are:

- Milk with a pinch of cardamom

- Clarified butter - Also called ghee, clarified butter has special properties that help decrease pitta – even though ghee is oily.
- Steamed broccoli
- Sunflower seeds
- Lassi (1/2 cup plain yogurt and ½ cup cumin-flavored water)
- Leafy greens and salads
- Cucumber
- Cold cereal
- Legumes and lentils
- Kichari (with coriander, fresh cilantro, and cumin)

Kapha benefits from light, hot and dry food. Some of the best kapha foods are:

- Warm rye, millet, or buckwheat
- Hot water with lemon, honey, and fresh ginger - In general, kapha does best with less food and the ginger-honey-lemon infusion can substitute for food.
- Astringent fruit like persimmon, apricot and pomegranate
- Kichari - Make it spicy with chili, pepper and fresh ginger.
- Leafy greens like beet greens, kale and dandelion
- Soymilk
- Sprouts
- Artichoke, green beans and cauliflower
- Legumes and lentils
- Brussels sprouts (steamed)

Everyone has the three doshas in them, just one or two is/are more dominant. However, there are certain foods that every body type can enjoy. These include:

- Kichari
- Mung dal
- Basmati rice
- Green beans and asparagus
- Berries, apricots, apples
- Clarified butter
- Cilantro and peas
- Goat's milk
- Sunflower seeds
- Lassi (1/2 cup plain yogurt and ½ cup water with a pinch of coriander, ginger, and cumin)

Kichari

You may notice that kichari is a mainstay among all the foods to eat for the vata, pitta and kapha types. Why? Kichari is an Ayurveda dish, which is mainly used during and after panchakarma (detox procedures) or illness. It is also used during healing fasts and it's a healing, perfectly balanced food for the three doshas.

It's best to use organic ingredients, and you can consume kichari – if you prefer it – on a two- to three-week monofast diet. Kichari can harmonize the mind and body and regulate your blood chemistry.

Ingredients:

- 1 to 2 tablespoons ghee (clarified butter) or any healthy cooking oil
- ½ cup basmati rice
- 1 cup mung beans (yellow split beans or green whole mung beans)
- 2 teaspoons coriander, ground
- 1 teaspoon turmeric, ground

- 1 teaspoon each of fenugreek seeds, mustard seeds, and cumin seeds
- 1 to 3 teaspoons fresh ginger, grated
- 1/8 teaspoon of asafetida or hing (optional)
- 6 to 8 cups water
- Organic vegetables (your choice). You can use any vegetables except onions, garlic, tomatoes, bell peppers, potatoes, and eggplant.

Rinse the rice and mung beans three times before cooking. Soak the beans one to eight hours. The process can help in eliminating gas formation.

In a deep pot over low to medium heat, melt the ghee or your choice of quality cooking oil. Add the grated ginger, mustard seeds, fenugreek and cumin. Sauté until slightly browned and not burnt.

Add the drained mung beans and rice and sauté for about 30 seconds more. Lower the heat. Add the hing, coriander and turmeric powders and sauté for 30 more seconds.

Add the water. The kitchari must be of soup consistency, so add more water as your see fit. Add the organic root vegetables. Cover the pot and simmer for 20 to 30 minutes. Add leafy greens. Cook further for 20 minutes more.

Serve. If you desire, add a little salt on top or Bragg's seasoning.

--

The world is your table. As long as you know the basic foods to eat for your dosha type and are familiar with the six tastes, you will know other kinds of food that belong to a certain taste even if they are not listed above. While the Ayurveda diet only requires you to follow a few simple rules, it is still important to learn more about the six tastes. Once you are already familiar with them, losing weight or attaining optimal health will be relatively easy.

Chapter 4: Losing Weight through Ayurveda

Mind and body balance in the Ayurveda diet take precedence over weight loss. However, if you want to lose weight through Ayurveda, know that you are overweight probably because your kapha dosha is not balanced. It's also important to know that your body has the three dosha types, with one or two dominating others. In Ayurveda, the kapha dosha may be helped through dietary intervention.

Ayurveda claims that individuals prone to the kapha dosha have low digestive fire, and they should do away with consuming heavy meals. People having low digestive fire should consume lighter meals, instead. Those who are predominantly kapha should limit eating sour, salty and sweet foods that call for high digestive fire to digest.

If you are predominantly kapha, increase your intake of pungent, astringent or bitter foods that promote digestive enzyme secretion. Consuming cold foods and beverages may aggravate the kapha dosha. Kapha people should not also eat too quickly or too slowly. Eating at a high or slow pace may prompt a person to overeat.

Excess in Kapha Dosha

In Ayurveda, being overweight entails an excess of kapha dosha. While it may not be the sole factor in dealing with excess weight, kapha certainly plays an important role.

One of Ayurveda's main principles is that opposites balance and like increases like.

Excess weight and kapha have similar attributes. Both of them slow, heavy, smooth, oily, cool, soft, dense, gross and stable, thus, being overweight can provoke the body's kapha. Excess body kapha can lead to obesity. On the contrary, achieving balance entails a surge in opposing influences like sharp, light, dry, hot, liquid, rough, subtle and mobile.

The Ayurveda diet does not center on short-term gains, so you don't need to starve yourself deliberately, or limit the food variety you can enjoy unrealistically. With the Ayurveda diet, you can follow a time-tested and clear path to excellent health.

When you are trying to lose weight through the Ayurveda diet, you may consider committing to follow five simple steps to help you reach your desired weight.

- Do yoga for 15 minutes every morning.

- Eat three satiating meals every day.

- Adhere to a kapha pacifying diet.

- Exercise for a minimum of three days a week.

- Set a daily routine to support your weight loss commitments.

The commitments are intuitive and simple. While you may have to exercise discipline in the beginning, your body's inherent intelligence will soon resurface with balanced urges in place of unhealthy cravings. When you attain such balance, sticking to your commitments gets easier until you notice that they are already becoming second nature.

One of the book's important topics is losing weight through the Ayurveda diet. Below are pointers on following the kapha pacifying diet. As mentioned earlier, an excess of kapha leads to obesity. If you feel that you are overweight, you may have to know more about the kapha pacifying diet.

Kapha Pacifying Diet

Kapha balance is attained by eating a diet rich in whole, freshly-cooked foods that are dry, light, well-spiced, relatively easily digestible and warming. Such foods are best served hot or warm. The foods normalize kapha by regulating moisture levels, balancing mucus production, maintaining sufficient heat and supporting elimination and proper digestion.

As kapha is naturally substantive, the right diet is one of the most efficient ways to achieve your desired weight. Kapha calls for a minimalistic diet with small quantities, fewer sweets, little snacking or none, various legumes, an abundance of fresh vegetables and fruits and minimal to no alcohol.

Qualities to Avoid and Favor

Kapha is smooth, oily, cool and heavy. Eating foods to neutralize kapha qualities (foods that are rough, dry, warm and light) can help to normalize kapha.

Favor airy and light over heavy and dense. Vegetables and fruit are light, thus, a diet based on fresh fruits and vegetables (cooked) is a great way to begin the kapha pacifying diet. Kapha is also balanced by raw vegetables and salads when they are in season. Black and green teas are preferable over the heavier coffee.

In general, avoid heavy foods like puddings, hard cheeses, cakes, nuts, wheat, pies, pastas, bread, most flours, deep fried foods, and red meat. Overeating at one sitting also causes heaviness. Avoid processed foods and heavy meals as they aggravate kapha's heaviness.

Favor warm over cold or cool. Eat foods with a warming energy. This means you need to utilize heating spices. Fortunately, spices are naturally warming and nearly all of them balance the kapha. Cooked foods are easily digestible and offer a warmer energy. Especially during the colder months, drink only hot, warm, or room temperature beverages. Conversely, avoid cooling energetic foods, frozen and cold drinks or food, leftovers from the refrigerator, and carbonated drinks.

Favor dry over oily or moist. The oiliness of kapha is offset by drying foods like popcorn, rice cakes, dried fruits, white potatoes, beans, and the rare glass of white or red wine. When cooking, use oil sparingly. You also need to minimize or eliminate foods like coconut, avocado, buttermilk, olives, eggs, cheese, cow's milk, eggs, nuts, seeds, and wheat. Kapha can easily retain water, so you must not drink water or liquids to excess. Moreover, avoid moist foods like summer squash, melons, yogurt, and zucchini, all of which can provoke kapha.

Favor rough over smooth. Vegetables and fruits' fibrous structure lends them a rough quality. Vegetables and fruits are easily digestible when cooked, but you should avoid overcooking them. Certain foods like cauliflower, cabbage, broccoli, many beans and dark leafy greens are high in roughage and can counteract kapha's oily, smooth nature. However, eating smooth foods like rice pudding, bananas, milk, hot cereal and cheese, can rapidly aggravate kapha.

Tastes to Avoid and Favor

Kapha is aggravated by the salty, sour and sweet tastes and is pacified by the bitter, astringent and pungent tastes. Understanding the tastes enables you to navigate the diet without constantly referring to lists of foods to avoid and favor.

Remember to emphasize pungent, bitter and astringent tastes. Minimize or avoid sweet, sour and salty tastes.

Eating to Balance Kapha

How you eat can impact your success when it comes to pacifying kapha. To balance kapha, you may want to eat three meals daily and eat those meals consistently. There are others who say that two meals are sufficient. You can also jumpstart a slow digestive fire (agni) for about 30 minutes before dinner and lunch by chewing ginger with a few lime juice drops, a pinch of salt, and ¼ teaspoon honey.

Excess bread, sweets and fast food can provoke kapha. You can lessen such foods' detrimental potential by ensuring they are served warm, taken sparingly, and are seasoned with warming spices and herbs. As kapha digestion is somewhat sluggish, you can also benefit with periodic cleanses or fasts. A short juice or fruit fast or a kichari monofast may help in the weight loss process.

Chapter 5: Food Combinations to Avoid

The topic applies to all dosha types. The combination of food is a health-conscious eating approach, wherein foods needing different digestive environments are separately consumed. While food combination theories may have controversial views, there are certain points that such theories agree on.

There are some food combinations that Ayurveda, physiologists, and contemporary hygienists consider bad. Some consequences from following bad food combos are problems with elimination, fatigue, nausea, stomachache, bloating, gas and digestive discomfort.

While the short-term effects of bad food combinations disappear within one day or two, long-term practices may lead to more severe issues like dry skin, bad breath, chronic inflammation, rashes, low energy, chronic digestion issues, and poor sleep. Many people naturally lose weight and feel an energy surge once they become mindful of the following food combination pitfalls.

Grilled cheese sandwich or lasagna. Starch-protein food combinations inhibit starch's salivary digestion. Starches and proteins require different acidity levels and different enzymes to be digested. When you eat starch and protein together, you force your body to digest protein and not starches.

A proponent of natural hygiene ideas, Dr. Herbert Shelton, states that undigested starchy food goes through decomposition and fermentation. In time, it leads to toxic end-products. It is much easier to add greens to cheesy dishes, as the stomach can easily digest them.

Fruit after a meal. It is considered that fruit does not combine well with other kinds of food, because it has simple sugars that don't need digestion. Thus, fruits do not stay long in your stomach.

Since they need more time to digest, foods like starchy, protein-rich and fatty foods will stay longer in the stomach. If you eat fruit after a meal, its sugar will ferment if it stays long in the stomach.

Meat and cheese omelet. Protein/protein combos are generally not suggested. A single protein source per meal won't need a lot of energy and is easier to digest. Eat a vegetable omelet, instead.

Cheese and tomato pasta sauce. Tomatoes are deemed acidic and should not be mixed with starchy carbohydrates. The theory calls for the avoidance of mixing acidic foods with carbohydrates. With the addition of dairy, you may encounter after-eating fatigue and digestive issues as your body will need a lot of energy to digest the meal. Eat your pasta with grilled vegetables and pesto, instead.

Oatmeal or cereal with orange juice and milk. Acid in acidic fruit or orange juice destroys the enzyme for digesting the starches in cereal. Acidic juices and fruits can also thicken milk and turn it into a mucus-forming, heavy substance. For a nutritious breakfast, have your juice or fruit half an hour before eating oatmeal.

Prosciutto and melon. Eat melons alone. The same applies for all fruits high in sugar. Generally, you need to eat fruits separately from starches or proteins, particularly if you want an instant energy surge from a fruit.

Cheese and beans. A common combination in Mexican cuisine is beans and dairy protein. Eaten with hot sauce and guacamole, a cheese-been combination is nearly guaranteed to lead to bloating and gas. Beans, by themselves, do not cause bloat; the food combo does. If you are detoxing your body or have weak digestion, skip the tomatoes and the cheese.

Yogurt with fruit. In Ayurveda, don't mix dairy with sour fruits as such combination can change the intestinal flora, diminish digestive fire, produce toxins and even cause allergies, cough, cold and sinus congestion. Ayurveda suggests the avoidance of digestive and congestive fire-dampening foods, like fruits mixed into cold yogurt.

If you still want to have that yogurt parfait, you can make it more digestion-friendly. Have an unflavored, room temperature yogurt. Instead of sour berries, add raisins, cinnamon and honey to the yogurt.

Milk and bananas. Such combination is considered in Ayurveda as toxin-forming and heavy. The combination is believed to slow down the mind and create heaviness within the body. If you can't avoid such combo, ensure that you are using ripe banana. Also, add nutmeg and cardamom to facilitate easy digestion.

Lemon dressing on tomato and cucumber salad. Nightshades like tomatoes, eggplant, chilies and potatoes should not be combined with cucumbers. Lemon also does not go well with such foods.

Chapter 6: Other Eating Rules to Consider

Ayurveda can be considered a lifestyle, and an effective way to normalize weight. It also offers great eating guides, particularly when it comes to digestion. The following are some Ayurveda guidelines (that apply to all doshas) that you should aim to follow.

Eat only when hungry. It means you should be truly hungry, and your previous meal has been digested completely. There are times when you may think that you are hungry, but you are actually just dehydrated. Adapt to your body's rhythm and find out what true hunger is.

Eat the appropriate quantity. Everybody is different, with various metabolic speeds, stomach sizes and needs. Listen to what your body signals to you and only eat until you feel fully satisfied.

Eat quality food. Ensure that your meal is a little oily or juicy as it can help improve nutrient absorption and promote digestion. Avoid foods that are too dry.

Eat warm meals. It's ideal to eat foods that are freshly cooked. As long as you don't eat anything directly from the refrigerator, you can preserve your *Agni* (digestive power). Eating warm foods enables your digestive enzymes to function efficiently.

Be mindful when you're eating. Rely on all your senses. Appreciate how your plate looks, your meal's aroma, your food's texture, the various flavors, and the sounds you make and hear as you eat.

<u>Don't eat conflicting food items together</u>. You may be risking an upset stomach.

<u>Eat at regular hours</u>. Nature likes regularity and cycles, so you should follow.

In, it is important to emphasize proper digestion and the right metabolism of food. When properly followed, the Ayurveda diet can help you become healthier, stave off various diseases, and lose weight. One of the most important things you can do for your health is to eat properly and wisely.

Just like medicine, food is considered powerful. There is even a *sloka* (ancient Ayurveda text writing) that says, 'food is medicine when properly consumed.' If you eat foods that are specific to your physiology, and adhere to a life-supporting (sattvic) routine, which promotes proper digestion, your body can surely benefit.

Eventually, you will discover that you will be healthier, happier and feel revitalized. When you properly stick to the Ayurveda diet, you will lose weight and normalize it. In Ayurveda, you metabolize with all your five senses, and you don't only metabolize food.

Everything you taste, smell, see, touch and hear becomes a part of you, thus, you should live a healthier life (and a fitter one) by making wiser food and life choices.

Conclusion

Thank you again for downloading this book!

I hope this book was able to help you to know more about the principles of Ayurveda when it concerns diet and weight loss.

The next step is to understand the Ayurveda diet more through research. After fully grasping the principles of Ayurveda and its dietary principles, you can now buy the food items you need to lose weight successfully. This is possible by adhering to the ancient Indian system's dietary principles.

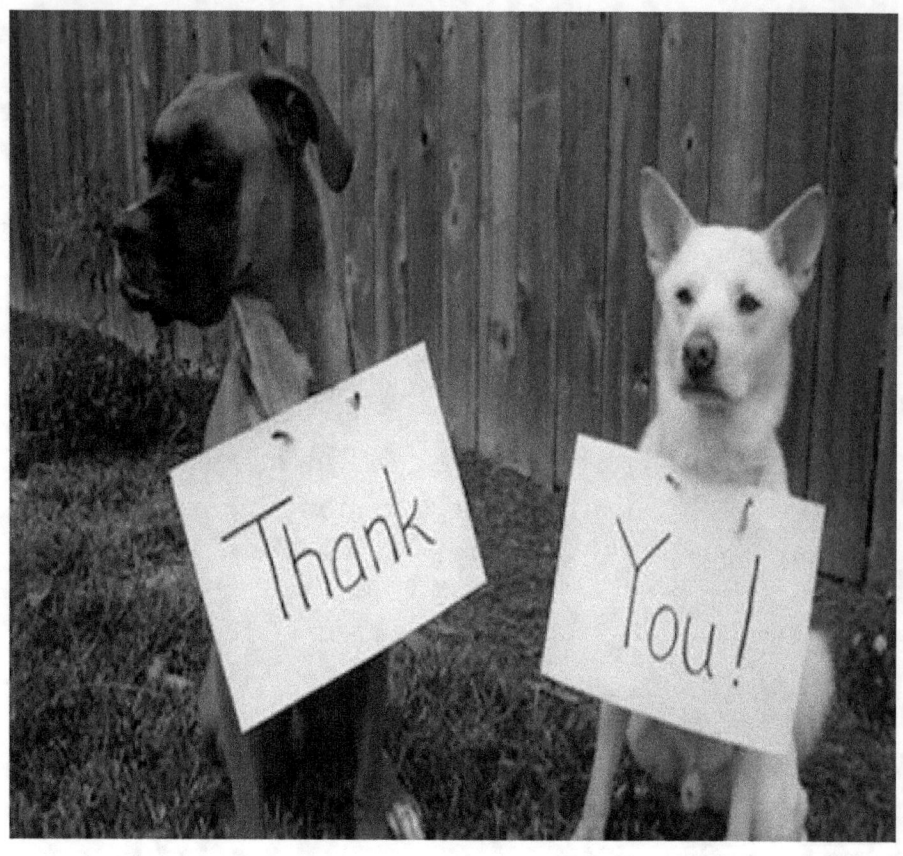

Finally, if you enjoyed this book, then I'd like to ask you for a favor, would you be kind enough to leave a review for this book on Amazon? It'd be greatly appreciated!

Thank you and good luck!

www.ingramcontent.com/pod-product-compliance
Lightning Source LLC
Chambersburg PA
CBHW061939280526
45787CB00004B/1657